Big bea [barcode: D0997960]

I have ♡ meeting you & my Jonathan

THE BLOKE'S 100 TOP TIPS FOR SURVIVING PREGNANCY

Dove for you is feelin tearfully massive & will grow for many a year to come - have fun tonight, Aarron!

oops sp@13!

love Nicky x

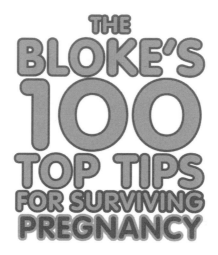

Jon Smith

HAY HOUSE

Australia • Canada • Hong Kong
South Africa • United Kingdom • United States

First published and distributed in the United Kingdom by Hay House UK Ltd, 292B Kensal Rd, London W10 5BE. Tel.: (44) 20 8962 1230; Fax: (44) 20 8962 1239. www.hayhouse.co.uk

Published and distributed in the United States of America by Hay House, Inc., PO Box 5100, Carlsbad, CA 92018-5100. Tel.: (1) 760 431 7695 or (800) 654 5126; Fax (1) 760 431 6948 or (800) 650 5115. www.hayhouse.com

Published and distributed in Australia by Hay House Australia Ltd, 18/36 Ralph St., Alexandra NSW 2015. Tel.: (61) 2 9669 4299; Fax: (61) 2 9669 4144. www.hayhouse.com.au

Published and distributed in the Republic of South Africa by Hay House SA (Pty), Ltd, PO Box 990, Witkoppen 2068. Tel./Fax: (27) 11 706 6612. orders@psdprom.co.za

Distributed in Canada by Raincoast, 9050 Shaughnessy St., Vancouver, BC V6P 6E5. Tel.: (1) 604 323 7100; Fax: (1) 604 323 2600

© Jon Smith, 2006

The author of this book does not dispense medical advice or prescribe the use of any technique as a form of treatment for physical or medical problems without the advice of a physician, either directly or indirectly. The intent of the author is only to offer information of a general nature to help you in your quest for emotional and spiritual well-being. In the event you use any of the information in this book for yourself, which is your constitutional right, the author and the publisher assume no responsibility for your actions.

A catalogue record for this book is available from the British Library.

ISBN 1-4019-0792-X
ISBN 978-1-4019-0792-1

Design: Leanne Siu
Printed and bound in Great Britain

DEDICATION

To Lisa –
Thank you for continuing to put up with an eejit

To Alia and Ronin –
Thank you for being the most beautiful
children in the world

ABOUT THE AUTHOR

Jon Smith lives in Spain with his wife Lisa, and their children Alia and Ronin. Jon writes fiction, non-fiction, books for children and musical theatre. His column *Dear Dad...* appears in *FQ* magazine.

Contact the Author

By post:
Jon Smith
c/o Hay House UK
292B Kensal Road
London W10 5BE

By e-mail:
jon@blokesguide.com

Websites of Interest:
http://www.blokesguide.com
http://www.hayhouse.co.uk

CONTENTS

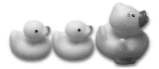

PREFACE

Pregnancy really is a scary word for us blokes. No matter how much we want to have children, when the news is confirmed, we get scared. Our fear isn't irrational, or a sign of weakness and therefore proof of our unsuitability as fathers. Far from it, some fear is healthy – it means we are involved emotionally with what is going on around us and inside our partner's body. We're scared of a lot of things, not least the unknown. Will our baby be healthy? Will our partner be all right? Will I be OK? Thankfully, you'll all get through this, one way or another. Pregnancy can also be a lot of fun, if you know what to expect. It's nice to be prepared.

You may be wondering why I called this *The Bloke's Top Tips for Surviving Pregnancy* – after all, what is there for a bloke to survive? Surely it's the poor woman who has to go through all of the physical stresses and strains? And there's many a woman who would happily clip you round the ear for even suggesting that pregnancy is as trying a time for the blokes as it is for the girls? But even though it's different for us, it's still an emotional roller-coaster – I hope these tips will help you through some of the highs and lows.

The 100 tips are set out roughly in the chronological order in which you'll need them. I've divided them into the three trimesters – each trimester lasts roughly three months. Some tips you will use, others you won't. The pregnancy your partner is experiencing is as unique as you are, and as unique as the child she is carrying. Do what you feel is right at any given time – because it probably is right. Refer to this book as and when you need to. These tips are mainly there as guidance, so you don't make the same fateful mistakes as those who have gone before you.

So, how do you use this book? Dip in, dip out or read it from start to finish in one sitting. It really doesn't matter. Most importantly, enjoy your partner's pregnancy and enjoy your new baby – who is only a matter of weeks away …

Good Luck and Congratulations!

Jon Smith

THE FIRST TRIMESTER

Tip 1

Taking It Like a Man

Not everyone reacts positively to such life-changing news. No matter what your immediate reaction is (how about 'Help!'), try not to respond negatively. It would be more worrying if you weren't worried – it's a blooming big life change. In a strange way, worrying is a sign that you've taken on the enormity of the change ... you've just created a new life! Think before you speak and remember that worrying can actually be positive – it can help you focus on the task at hand and prepare you for fatherhood.

Tip 2

For Those Who Are over the Moon

Well done. The result has come through. You knew you could do it – and you were right! Enjoy that elation and don't let anyone rain on your parade. Be proud and start preparing yourself for what is to come in the next few months. The pregnancy may be hard on you both, but whatever you do, don't ever let on to your wife that you're suffering as much as she is! Moving forward in a positive frame of mind is going to make things easier all round.

Tip 3

The Fear

No matter how scared, worried or downright petrified you are about the birth of your child, know that it will all be OK. You're not the first and you certainly won't be the last to be reduced to a quivering wreck by the prospect of impending fatherhood. You *can* afford this baby; and yes, your car *is* suitable, as is your house or flat. You *will* be able to change a nappy and bath a child. Life as you know it will not end once the baby is born (although you might spend a lot more time in the park than you did before).

Fear of the unknown is completely logical and natural. You might feel that you are about to spontaneously combust – but remember that these emotions hit thousands of people every week. They all survive. The fear will pass.

Tip 4

Morning (Noon and Night) Sickness

Many women experience 'morning sickness' during the early weeks of pregnancy (though the label is misleading as it can strike at any time of day). It's due to all the pregnancy hormones swilling around your partner's body and there really isn't a lot that you can do to help, although offering to clean up the mess and giving sensitive back rubs will be very much appreciated. Oh, and hold off asking for a night of unbridled passion – there's absolutely no chance, mate. It really isn't your cooking. Promise.

However, although morning sickness is one of the biggest clichés of pregnancy, along with bizarre food cravings, there are some women who never get sick. So don't worry if your partner doesn't experience any of these symptoms. Every pregnancy is unique.

Tip 5

Telling Your Mates

Best said man to man, which is a fantastic excuse for a great night out. However, don't expect your mates to be particularly helpful or supportive. Their reaction may well be one of pity rather than celebration. Nod and smile to all the predictable references to dirty nappies and no sleep. You know they love you, really.

Tip 6

Telling Your Parents

More than likely your parents will be over the moon with the news of a grandchild. However, be prepared – sometimes the shock of a first grandchild can be overwhelming. Be sensitive to the fact that your news can be hard-hitting – you are confirming that they are getting older and you have finally grown up, all with one simple sentence. When they do get used to the idea, you will be swamped with gifts and advice, some useful:

'Keep baby warm with lots of layers …'

and some not:

'A good smack to keep them in line; it didn't do you any harm.'

Tip 7

Telling Your Siblings

Be prepared for some jealousy. If you are the first to have a child, you may inadvertently cause them to reassess their lives. If they have children too, then you are now in an ongoing competition with them as regards your child's ability, looks and temperament. Look out for the signs from the moment you announce the news:

'Well, little Philip was walking at seven days, which is very advanced.'

'Yes, and for Charlie's second birthday he insisted we go to the opera.'

'Due in December? Sagittarius? Lovely. They can be right little monsters, you know.'

Tip 8

Reacting to the In-Laws

Whether you regard relations with your in-laws to be good or bad, you'll have won a new level of respect with the news of a grandchild. You have now officially gone from defiler to family man. Wallow in this new-found respect. Might even be a good time to ask for some money for home improvements …

Tip 9

....

Telling Your Boss

Assuming that you will not let the cat out of the bag until after the twelve-week 'embargo' (once you're past this milestone, and are into the second trimester, the risk of miscarriage is greatly reduced), it's well worth using your unborn child as a bargaining chip to improve your situation at work. You might be able to secure a pay rise, a change of hours and possibly even a promotion, if you negotiate your position well enough. If it's possible, look to maybe securing one day a week based at home. Not only is this extra time with your child and your partner, which is good for both relationships, it's also one less day of commuting.

Tip 10

Who's Going to Support Me?

No one. Your partner will be consumed with the baby growing inside her and will be bringing new meaning to the expression 'tired and emotional'. Your mates are scared that one of them will be next. Your parents think you're too irresponsible to have your own car/mortgage/pet – let alone a child – and your siblings just laugh at you. Take a deep breath and accept that you're on your own.

Tip 11

Feeling Fruity

Confirmation that you are both fertile and have impregnated your partner is a wonderful ego stroke. Watch you don't begin to alter your walk into a swagger and certainly ensure that you don't gyrate your hips in public – no matter how strong your desire.

Tip 12

So, Do You Want a Boy or a Girl?

If you have a personal preference for one gender over another, keep it very quiet. Unless you want a baby girl. It's safer that way. Trust me.

Tip 13
....

More Tests than an International Cricket Team

A modern-day pregnancy is a very public affair. Once your partner's doctor has confirmed the pregnancy, the next nine months will mean a miasma of tests, scans, appointments and visits. No matter how difficult it is to arrange time off, no matter how you feel about witnessing your partner being prodded and poked like a prize pig, be there for her as often as you can.

Most of the tests will be routine, although you may also have to make decisions about whether or not you both want to test for certain disorders. Whatever happens, your support will be hugely welcome. It's all about being involved with the pregnancy. And let's face it, even hospital waiting rooms can be far more entertaining than taking phone calls from aggrieved clients reminding you that you were supposed to send them a catalogue two weeks ago.

Tip 14

Scans

The ultrasound scan will be the first opportunity you have to see your baby. While most hospitals might be lacking glorious Technicolor, it's a wonder to behold. Don't miss out. And don't try to laminate the scan photo – it's printed on thermal paper and will turn completely black.

Tip 15

....

Seeing Red …?

The appearance of some blood (known as spotting) during pregnancy is very common and most likely to occur during the first twelve weeks of pregnancy. Although worrying, it does not necessarily mean something bad is happening. Try not to think the worst, but do encourage your partner to get a check-up with her doctor or midwife. In fact, in any situation where either of you are worried, it's always best to get checked out. This is one situation where you won't be made to feel like a silly child for wasting doctor's time.

Tip 16

Gen up!

Do make the effort to read up on pregnancy, labour, birth and the early years. Not only will you win countless brownie points, you will also be better equipped to deal with the events that are happening right now. Knowledge is power, my friend.

One good way is to subscribe to a website such as http://www.babycentre.co.uk where you can get the weekly low-down on your baby's development. All you need to know is your baby's due date and the information will come flooding in. Reading about pregnancy on the Net is also a great way to waste an entire afternoon at work, if you can get away with it.

Tip 17

Too Much to Take in?

However, you might as well accept that you will not become an expert on pregnancy during the next nine months. Or the next nine years, come to think of it. No one is expecting you to become a guru, just to take an active role in supporting your partner by asking the right questions and making constructive comments.

Do ask:
'Is it this week that the fingernails begin to develop?'

Don't ask:
'Once the baby is born, can I nip off to the World Cup for a few weeks?'

Tip 18

Will I Be a Good Dad?

If you want to, you will. There are no rulebooks or manuals that come with children. You will be able to cope and nothing is too hard, even changing nappies. Treat your child as you would like to be treated yourself and you will be a good dad – just don't force your idea of fashionable clothes (or music) on the poor innocent.

Tip 19

Is It Still OK to Go out with Friends?

Certainly not without permission! If that sounds a bit harsh, remember that if you're finding this pregnancy business a bit scary, imagine what's going through her mind, and she can't even escape down the pub for a night of drunken oblivion. Most of the time she will need you at home, with her. Sometimes, however, she might just want a girlie night in with a soppy video, or some friends, in which case you'll probably be granted shore leave.

But ultimately, your social life should and will take a nosedive during your partner's pregnancy. Cheer up, at least it's all good practice for the reality of life with a newborn.

Tip 20

Cravings

Most probably your partner will latch on to a certain foodstuff during her pregnancy. No matter what her poison, be sure to always have lots of whatever it is to hand. Know where to find the local supplier, should stocks suddenly be depleted from a night of overindulgence. Let's just hope she wants ice cream and not beluga caviar. Note that her craving may well suddenly change to something else without warning … and no matter how bizarre it may seem to you, do take that craving seriously!

Tip 21

Will Sex Hurt My Unborn Baby?

Not unless you really are hung like a donkey, rather than just thinking you are. Sex with your partner will not harm the baby physically or emotionally – although it might take you some time to get used to having three in the bed. (And with a rather different kind of threesome from the one usually featured in your fantasies ...)

Tip 22

No Sex

If sex doesn't seem to be on the agenda with the frequency it once was, it really isn't the end of the world – although it might feel like it. She's exhausted, already feeling invaded, and quite happy just to go to sleep. Sorry, big boy, but prodding and poking her all night will not have the desired effect. If it's any consolation, things will get better. Eventually.

Tip 23

Too Much Sex

And you're worried about this? It's not that uncommon for a woman's libido to increase during pregnancy, especially during the second trimester, a happy side-effect that can last until she simply becomes too big in the third trimester. If you are a man lucky enough to be enjoying this increase in sexual relations, perform your duty, enjoy your partner, but please don't rub it in. We're not all as lucky.

THE SECOND TRIMESTER

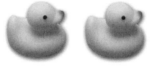

Tip 24

Weekend away

Congratulations, you've made it through the first three months, the morning sickness has probably subsided and you've no doubt 'gone public' with your news. Now's a good time to treat yourself and your partner to a night or two in a hotel – you won't get the opportunity again in a long while. Well, not with just the two of you in the bed, anyway. And by this stage your partner won't be so big and uncomfortable that a night or two of passion is out of the question. Go anywhere; it doesn't matter. Long hot bath (for her), minibar (for you) and a long lie-in for you both … bliss.

Tip 25

Watching the Wonderful Body-Morphing Process

Pregnancy is a total body experience. You will appreciate the larger bum and breasts; but were you really expecting the bigger feet, swollen hands and longer hair? Your baby is taking control of your partner and while beautiful, it can also be positively scary. This is all completely natural and healthy. Be sensitive. (Don't forget how self-critical most women are. Whatever physical changes you have noticed, she has already not only noticed but also studied in close-up and analysed in detail for more hours than bears thinking about – maybe this isn't the best time to re-introduce her to your Sid the Sexist jokes …)

Tip 26

Stretch Marks

The changing shape of your partner's body takes its toll on your partner's skin. The sudden increase in size, especially around her tummy, may mean the appearance of stretch marks – all completely normal and healthy. These little red lines won't go away but will fade to silver over time. Tell her you've hardly noticed them. Tell her you love her anyway …

Tip 27

You Banker!

It's time to knock the Tuesday night pub visits on the head. Not only will you save the money, you'll have one less headache a week, be more productive on a Wednesday and be able to buy something for the baby on a Saturday. Financial management starts here, and won't end until the bump is at least 21 years old. Your DVD collection will suffer; but don't worry, in a few months' time you won't have the time, or the energy, to be able to manage an entire film in one sitting, anyway.

Tip 28

....

Getting down with the DIY

Those jobs have been waiting to be done since the day you moved in. No more excuses! Painting can be quite good fun, honest. It really isn't as boring or difficult as it sounds – and think of the smug, overwhelming feeling of achievement you'll have when you've finished. And consider how many photos are going to be taken of the newborn … do you really want that flaky paint and bad wallpaper to be captured forever on camera?

Tip 29

Keep Your Cool

I'm sure you're always a calm and collected individual, but if there are occasions where you're likely to vent your spleen to your partner, think twice – she's on an emotional test-tube of hormones at the moment and something small and petty can quickly become something catastrophic. She may nag, moan, complain and mope around the place … ignore it. It's time to grow a thicker skin.

Tip 30

....

Listen up!

Everything about this pregnancy is exciting for your partner. It is for you too, but she will most likely want to talk about it, constantly. Listen to what she has got to say. A baby – your baby – is growing inside her, right now. How bizarre is that?

Tip 31

....

To Move, or not to Move

Moving house is a pretty stressful event at the best of times. Throw a pregnancy into the mix and you're in for a real experience. However, if you do need to move to make your home environment more suitable for the arrival of a little one, jump in with both feet. Put your house on the market immediately. You need to be established in your new home with weeks, if not months, to spare before baby's arrival.

Tip 32

Refrigerate This!

No matter how large your fridge is now, you need a new one. Sorry, but your current one just won't do. Just where exactly do you plan to put the vast array of prepared food for your weaning infant? Your fridge will no longer be the well-stocked minibar it was once; prepare to meet the chilled food store of vegetable gloop greatness.

Tip 33
....

When Was the Last Time You Washed That?

It's also time to say goodbye to the launderette, once and for all. With a new baby about to appear, think of all the bibs, babygros, clothes, blankets, sheets of muslin, and of course your own puke-sodden garments that will need a sound daily washing. Even if it has to take the place of the wall-mounted 32″ plasma screen in your lounge, you need a washing machine. Right now.

Tip 34

Bad Poo Days

Another of the many delights that a pregnant woman endures for the sake of furthering your genes is that her hormones may make her constipated. Sometimes for days on end. There's obviously not a tremendous amount you can do to help, other than be sensitive. What with everything else that's going on, she may not be in the mood for your lightning wit, or graphic descriptions of your own successful expulsion this morning.

Tip 35

Private Piles

Not drinking enough water, constipation and the baby depressing your partner's intestines can all help in the creation of haemorrhoids. You may be asked to apply certain creams to your partner's bum. A test of love and devotion, if ever there was one. As well as often popping up during pregnancy, piles can also put in an appearance during labour and delivery – well, hardly surprising when you think of all that straining …

Tip 36

Was That You?

Added to all these other indignities, don't be surprised if your partner suddenly starts passing wind in your presence for the first time in your relationship. It's completely normal; she can't help it, it's a by-product of the pregnancy. Let's face it, you'll still laugh.

Tip 37

Playing the Name Game

Take your time! Naming a child has a lifelong effect upon the beneficiary. Be kind, be original; accept ideas from others; but only ever settle on a name that makes both you and your partner smile when you say it out loud. Smile, that is, not laugh …

Tip 38

Preparing a Nursery

Although the baby will most probably be in a cot in your room for a number of months (yes, even if that means in your leather-walled bachelor shag pad), there will come a time when he or she will need their own space. Decorating a baby's room can be a lot of fun and is best done before your baby is born. Subtle colours, a few cuddly toys and a mobile are all you need for baby heaven.

Tip 39

On the Run

Although the extra time you're spending at home will be appreciated, it's best to maintain (or begin!) a healthy level of exercise throughout your partner's pregnancy. We've all heard of blokes having 'sympathetic pregnancies', but she's the one who's supposed to gain weight over the nine months – not you! In a few years' time you're going to have to run in the park with your growing child. You don't want to be beaten by a four-year-old, do you?

Tip 40

Don't Become Baby Obsessed

You will have long, long conversations about pregnancy and babies – and this is good. But be sure to take your own and your partner's mind off the baby once in a while. Try to get out to the cinema while you still can. Get out for meals and entertain friends. (Let your friends lead the conversation, though, otherwise within a matter of minutes you'll be talking about babies again.)

Tip 41

The Tears

Pregnant women cry. A lot. Sometimes it's your fault, but mostly it's her hormones wreaking havoc with her emotions. She won't know why she's crying and there's no way to predict likely causes. However, nappy adverts are usually a culprit.

Tip 42

Hello, My Dears

Big breasts throughout the pregnancy are fantastic. Even if you're not normally a 'breast man', you will stop in your tracks when you first appreciate the momentous physical change that has occurred. Enjoy them and let your partner know how much you enjoy them, although bear in mind that initially fondling them may be met with yelps of pain from your partner. Sadly, the Pamela Anderson effect will probably be gone once she stops breastfeeding …

Tip 43

Pantone

As well as her breasts growing to a magnificent size, your partner's nipples will also grow and become darker. Once she's finished breastfeeding, her nipples will return to their pre-pregnancy size along with her breasts. The new colour, however, is permanent.

Tip 44

Number Crunching

Your new role as a father means responsibility – especially in a financial sense. Use the focus of pregnancy to reassess how you are spending and look to reduce your debts as effectively as you can. Out with the shopping sprees and in with the saving. Time to be grown-up and seek financial advice. For instance, consolidation loans are often a sensible option and cheaper than paying off credit card companies. The more money you have to spend on your family, the better. Negotiating loans is as boring as it gets, but if you don't, it's your money you're wasting.

Tip 45

There Are Benefits to All This

Your homework today is to look into what benefits you are entitled to, both from the benevolent government of Her Majesty the Queen and from your employer. Legislation is always being altered, but you can look forward to paternity leave and child benefit – it's not a lot, but every little helps. After all, you've paid enough stamp over the past few years; and given that you will receive a pittance of a state pension, if at all, it's time you got some of it back.

Tip 46

Wedding Bells?

Your partner's pregnancy can cause you both to re-think of your domestic situation. It is still common for partners co-habiting, and expecting a child, to feel the time is right to get hitched, some out of propriety and some because they just feel it's the right thing to do. Only you know. Weddings are expensive. Best to get it done sooner rather than later, or wait until after the baby is born – at least then your partner will be able to wear the gorgeous dress and join in the celebratory champagne.

Tip 47

Where There's a Will ...

... your children and your partner are likely to benefit from the highly unlikely but minuscule chance that you are not long for this mortal plane. It's never easy to face up to death – but better to give your family the money than the state. Both you and your partner should make a will immediately, if you haven't done so already.

Tip 48

Thinking about Childcare?

Unless you're lucky enough to be loaded, you should be. Look into costs as soon as possible. Shop around. Childcare is hugely expensive and you must weigh up whether one of you will be working just to keep your child in nursery, or whether you'll be better off by both continuing to work. There are arguments for and against nurseries. Ignore them. Do what you both feel is right for you two and, of course, your baby.

Tip 49

When Daddy Is Mummy

These days there's far less of a social stigma to being a stay-at-home-dad. It's tremendously hard and you won't get paid, but believe it or not – and you won't until you do it – it is the most emotionally rewarding job in the world. Plus you'll get to hang out in parks with loads of women all day. Could be a viable option. Do think about it seriously, despite your ego, especially if your partner earns more than you.

Tip 50

Mum, Would You Mind?

If it's practical, it's well worth at least broaching the subject of either one of your parents or her parents looking after the little one during the day. With the outrageous cost of childcare, it is certainly a cheaper option. And how much more comfortable you will feel with a family member looking after your progeny than a paid stranger. But be prepared for them saying 'no' – after all, they've already had to go through the experience with you ...

Tip 51

Got a New Motor?

Out with the old and in with the new. Or, when you're expecting a baby, out with the racing-green-two-seater-babe-magnet and in with the new beige Volvo estate. Suits you, Sir. No, it really does.

Tip 52
....

Buying New Stuff

Don't be tempted to upgrade your DVD player, video recorder
or stereo. Stick with what you've got and make do. Everything
you own will be systematically trashed by your offspring
within the next two years. Slices of buttery toast and lasers
don't get on – trust me.

Tip 53

Who's the Twin Sister?

During the nine months of pregnancy you will be forgiven for thinking, on occasion, that you are living with your partner's twin sister. She looks the same and acts the same. But then, every now and again, she behaves ever so slightly different. Maybe your jokes aren't appreciated in the same way – your lightning wit is mistaken for sarcasm. Maybe a simple suggestion about which movie to rent becomes a full-blown argument about how unsupportive you've been recently. Who is this twin sister you're now sharing a house with? She's still your partner; but she's with baby and that's all there is to it. Tread with care.

Tip 54

....

The Moaning!

You might feel that in her opinion you can't do anything right. As far as she is concerned, you can't. Don't fight it; just accept that until the baby is born you are going to be picked on. A lot.

(Have some sympathy! As far as she's concerned, you're the one who got her into this mess in the first place ...)

Tip 55

Smelly!

However much you wash already, wash more. Wash to the point of developing an Obsessive Compulsive Disorder. Change your socks regularly. Brush your teeth five times a day. Even then, in her opinion, you will still stink. Sorry. Your partner's sense of smell is now incredibly sensitive and any slight pongs will be uncomfortable for her. Compensating with deodorants and aftershave won't do either – the chemical smells will be as off-putting as your 'natural odour'. You stinker.

Tip 56

What If I Don't Like It?

Worrying about your future relationship with your child is completely natural. Worry not, the moment your baby is born, you will fall instantly and unconditionally in love with the little mite. Even if he has ginger hair.

Tip 57

Sleep Monster

Your partner is tired, very tired. All the time, and not just of you! Fatigue is completely normal; apparently a woman's pregnant body is working harder even when she's resting than a non-pregnant body is when mountain-climbing – you just can't see the efforts. And that's not even to mention the emotional strain she's under ... So don't suggest a quick game of squash, but do suggest the occasional walk around the block. If you are inviting friends round for the evening, be prepared for your partner calling it a night at 8.30 or 9.00 pm. Right after she's told you off for something. Again.

Tip 58

She Snores

Yes, hello hormones and hello noisy nights. She's put up with you doing it for years, now it's payback time. Have a heart! It will stop when the baby is born. Or maybe not. Only time will tell.

Tip 59

It's Good to Talk

Once the bump is visible and the first kicks and punches are vibrating, you might feel the urge to talk to your baby. You'll feel a bit strange at first, but you're making the first bond with your child. It's great when they kick at the sound of your voice. No matter how strong the temptation, shy away from the feigned 'coochie-coochie-coo' baby voice and use only your normal manly tones – otherwise your baby won't know who you are when she eventually pops out – she'll be looking round for the cartoon character you sounded like for the past few months.

Tip 60

....

Sharing Tastes

From early on in the pregnancy, feel free to introduce your unborn child to the aural wonder of your music collection (and even your singing). Your baby will love it and respond accordingly. Familiar tunes may prove very useful after the birth, when you are trying to get your baby off to sleep. (And it doesn't have to be *Twinkle Twinkle Little Star* – Ice Cube's *War and Peace* was a big sleep-hit in our house.)

Tip 61

Making Yourself Useful

If you're feeling a bit left out of all the action, there's lots of jobs to be getting on with. All those new clothes and blankets the two of you are buying in for the baby need a wash before they can be used. Offer to do this – and while you're at it, maybe do a few loads of yours and your partner's clothes too. Who said it was her job, anyway? If you don't know how the washing machine works, feel very ashamed of yourself and ask. (A 40° wash is usually a safe bet.)

Tip 62

Learning New Skills

The same can be said for helping out more with the other domestic duties of the house. There're probably your shirts that need ironing and your dinner that needs cooking – don't be proud, chip in. The great thing about cooking is you get to decide what you're both eating. Although I'm not saying she will necessarily like it. See all that filth under your side of the bed – that's you, that is. Hair, skin, dirt … there's probably a dustpan and brush under the sink. Have a look.

Tip 63

Her Bum's Bigger

Say nothing! Absolutely nothing. It's much better not to tell the truth.

THE THIRD TRIMESTER

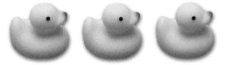

Tip 64

Planning the Birth

As the pregnancy lumbers into its final stretch and the end looms into sight, it's time to start planning for the main event. The Birth Plan is a document that lists your partner's preferences for labour and delivery. Most importantly, it will list her desired pain relief and preferred birth position.

By all means assist your partner with her birth plan – but do remember that it is her birth plan, not yours. Feel you can make suggestions only when you spot references that might be slightly unrealistic (she wants five eunuchs to throw rose petals on the newborn, catering requirements that wouldn't be out of place for a BBC film crew, and Dale Winton to compère the labour …). Understand why she is making the decisions she makes and support her. When the time comes, you will have to be her voice too.

Tip 65

....

Check It out

If you are given the opportunity to visit the hospital where your partner will be giving birth, try and go along. At least the place won't be a complete maze to you when you are there for real. Ask questions, get to know the layout and find out the number you should call when your partner is in labour. And write it down somewhere you won't forget. Like by the beer shelf in the fridge.

Tip 66

Route Planner

It is also a good idea to practise the route to the hospital, at various different times of the day, at weekends and on weekdays. All sense of direction will probably desert you when driving your partner to hospital in the full throes of labour. While you might know where the hospital is, do you know where the maternity unit is? Which door should you use at night? Better to have all this clear in your head now.

Tip 67

Come on!

You still haven't painted the walls, or finished building the shelves, have you? There's always something more pressing. You really must get a move on. It's not long now.

Tip 68

....

Keep an Eye out

Your partner may well decide to 'help' you out with some of the outstanding tasks left to be done. This is partly due to her wanting the place to be 'just right', but mainly due to frustration at your empty promises. Don't be surprised to come home to your partner struggling at the top of a loft ladder with drills, electric saws and nail guns. Take the hint.

Tip 69

Pack a Bag

Well worth having a bag of your own packed and ready to go (leave it in the car). Stock up on all your favourite snacks and fizzy drinks (not beer). Don't bring the *Gameboy* – that might be interpreted as very rude.

Tip 70

NCT Meetings

A bit strange, really, but well worth the money and the effort. The National Childbirth Trust offer courses throughout the country. Both for mums and dads-to-be, the courses provide you with the opportunity to meet others who will be having a baby about the same time. The men will be awkward and avoid eye contact, while the girls will be talking embarrassingly openly about everything intimate to do with childbirth. Bring your own Rich Tea, just in case.

Tip 71

....

NHS Antenatal Meetings

The raw, unabridged director's cut of pregnancy and childbirth. This is, quite simply, how it is. Too graphic to even warrant biscuits. Very useful, very honest and no ridiculous 'get to know each other's name' games.

Tip 72

Boy Nesting

Try as you might to resist it, you too will begin to clear out your old belongings, and generally make room for the new arrival. Not forgetting, of course, making room for the apparatus that accompanies a new arrival. Welcome to the world of car-boot sales.

Tip 73

Sex after Birth?

It's a sad indictment, but most men, if they think at all about what will happen *after* the birth, think about it in terms of their conjugal rights, rather than about any baby. Rest assured, you will be back in the 'driving seat', so to speak, at some stage after the birth. There's no fixed timescale; your partner will need to heal first, both physically and emotionally. Don't push it. And no, sex with your partner after she has given birth is not any different.

Tip 74

Tossed out of Bed

Towards the end of the pregnancy you might be ordered to leave the matrimonial bed. Your partner will be very sensitive to temperature, space and her share of the duvet. Your presence may simply no longer be welcome. Say hello to the sofa or the spare room. In fairness, you will probably get a better night's sleep, if a somewhat lonelier one.

Tip 75

Toying with Nature

One way to pass those interminable final few weeks is by mimicking the sound of a baby sucking, which will often result in your partner lactating. Highly amusing – for you, that is, not for your partner.

Tip 76

The Presence of Presents

To avoid feeling like a complete social pariah, I strongly suggest that you take a moment to arrange a 'birth present' for your partner for that all important first visit after all the drama has died down and the baby is born. It really doesn't matter what the gift is; just ensure that you arrive at the hospital with a 'special something' up your sleeve – or in your pocket. And no, a hanky won't do.

Tip 77

What a Drag

Despite your mutual excitement over the imminent arrival, you won't be the first to feel a bit bored towards the end. A watched kettle never boils, and nine months can suddenly feel like nine years. Chin up, it really will happen soon. However impatient you are, at least you're not the one having to waddle down the street with a two-stone egg inside your stomach. She will be rather keen for it all to be over too.

Tip 78

Don't Clock-Watch

If you're at work, eagerly awaiting the call to say she is in labour, don't clock-watch. The days will drag. The call will come, when it comes. Try to throw yourself into your work, to take your mind off it. Chances are, your baby will be born in the early hours of the morning, anyway. And certainly do not ask your partner when the baby is coming – she doesn't know either.

Tip 79

Phone List

Before you forget, write down the numbers of all those you will want to call to announce the birth. Do it now, or you will forget. Don't rely on your mobile phone's memory – chances are you'll forget to recharge your battery and it will run out. Some dads even prepare the text template in advance and just fill in the sex, weight and amount of hair after the event.

Tip 80

Contractions

Finally, when the time is right, your partner's womb will begin to contract – the process necessary to get baby out. These cramp-like, stabbing feelings are far, far worse than we can ever imagine. Yes, it will hurt and the pain will get progressively worse as the labour progresses. Offer back rubs and talk to your partner to keep her mind off the pain – it probably won't work, but you will prove to be a distraction, if nothing else.

Tip 81

The Show

The show is effectively the 'plug' keeping your baby in the womb. When your partner announces she has had a 'show' she is not referring to Andrew Lloyd Webber. Once the show has been passed, labour has not necessarily begun, but it won't be long now. Get that champagne on ice ...

Tip 82

The Breaking of the Waters

This is the one they always show happening in the most unlikely and dramatic places in the movies. Life is usually far more prosaic. Your partner's waters will break, either of their own accord, or with assistance from a midwife. Either way, you're really close now. Your baby will be born within the next 24 hours. Fact.

Tip 83

Induction

If none of the above events looks imminent, you and your partner won't be the only ones to become bored with the waiting game. Once the delivery date has been reached and breached, the doctors will be pretty impatient too. Thankfully, two weeks is your limit and then that baby is coming out, ready or not. Induction is particularly common in first births, and is a straightforward procedure involving hormones being given to kick-start labour. Think of it rather like a car being jump-started.

Tip 84

Caesarean Section

In an ideal world, your baby will be born 'naturally'. However, on occasion, a Caesarean section may be necessary. If you or your doctors have decided that this is the safest option, help your partner prepare for what is essentially major surgery. While the operation is now commonplace, it is still a scary prospect, mainly because she will be awake during the procedure. Take comfort from knowing that at a prescribed date and time your baby will be born. Your partner will be especially reliant on you after the birth as she will be incapable of moving around, lifting or driving, for at least a few weeks.

Tip 85

Breech Birth

Less likely now than ever before, with many expecting couples, midwives and doctors opting for Caesarean section. However, babies can be and are born in the breech position – which means feet (or buttocks), rather than head, first. It is quite possible, but obviously not anyone's first choice. Sore – but worth it.

Tip 86

TENS

Once contractions have kicked in, there are several different options for pain relief. Unless the medical staff need to intervene, your partner can choose which, if any, pain relief she requires. The entry-level option is a TENS machine. TENS machines consist of lots of wires, pads and a battery pack. The pads are placed around your partner's back and the electrical charges are supposed to ease the pain of the early stages of labour. Not only is it pretty useless, it gets in the way *and* you'll have to pay to hire one …

Tip 87

Entonox

Entonox is the posh term for gas and air. A firm favourite with the natural childbirth camp. Will do wonders for your nerves, if you steal a blast – but very little to ease your partner's discomfort. A lot of fuss about nothing, to be totally honest. But, it seems to work for some women.

Tip 88

....

Pethidine

Mind-altering drug, free of charge. You've got to love the NHS. Pethidine will affect your baby and make him very sleepy, but after the trauma of birth, who could blame him for wanting a few days' kip. It will also ease your partner's pain.

Tip 89

Epidural

This is the daddy of pain relief. Assuming the anaesthetist hits the spot, your partner will be paralysed (temporarily, of course) from the waist down. Other than having a needle stuck in her spinal column, she won't feel a thing. The downside is that an epidural can actually draw out labour, because your partner won't be able to push so effectively. But by this stage she's probably in such agony she's beyond caring, anyway ...

Tip 90

What not to Wear

Dress down; not just because it's a Friday but also because if hospitals are generally hot, then delivery suites are infernos. Go for the T-shirt and trouser combo. Generous with the deodorant and light on the aftershave, please (after all, it's a closed room). Oh, and comfortable footwear, if you will.

Tip 91

You Got Change for a Twenty?

At four in the morning, you'll be lucky to find anyone with any change in their pocket, full stop. Be prepared, change your notes into coins and you'll be armed for the car park, vending machine and public telephone (mobiles aren't allowed in hospital, they affect the navigational instruments).

Tip 92

....

The Birth

It's what this whole adventure has been all about. The baby is finally coming out! Whether the birth is assisted by surgery or medical instruments, is at home or in a hospital, is in water or on dry land – it doesn't matter. It's wonderful; the closest you'll ever get to a miracle. Overcome your squeamishness and enjoy it as much as you can.

Tip 93

Cutting the Cord

If you want to cut the cord – tell the midwife. Even if it's written in large red crayon on the birth plan. As you may come to notice, the document will probably have been completely ignored, anyway. Stand up for yourself, man, and let the midwife know. If you mention it before the birth, be sure to remind her, or it will be lopped off in the blink of an eye.

Tip 94

The Placenta

Labour is not over with the birth of your baby, believe it or not. The third stage of labour is the passing of the placenta or the afterbirth. This bizarre sack has been your baby's home for the last nine months and now needs to come out. Compared to the baby, it will be a doddle for your partner. Try not to faint when you see it. It looks very, very weird.

Tip 95

Feeling a Bit Weepy?

It's an emotional experience this having a baby lark. Nine months of angst and worry and concerns, and then, all of a sudden you're a dad. How did that happen? It might be about this time that you cry like a little girl who's had her hair pulled. You're excused. You big jessie.

Tip 96

A Moment Alone, Please?

There may well be a lot of people in the delivery room when the baby makes a first appearance. And this is a good thing. Don't worry if it all feels a little crowded; they'll be off to deliver another baby soon. Leaving you, your partner and your minutes-old baby a chance to get to know each other … Your jaw will be aching about now from the large grin that's been on your face since the birth. And you won't be the first, or last, to wonder how something can be so small and so big at the same time.

Tip 97

Who Do You Phone First?

Assuming that you have a list prepared, ignore it and phone your mum. Mums are great at passing on news and she will easily take care of 50 per cent of the list without you having to recharge your mobile or hang around outside for too long. Phone her parents next and then the grandparents. Lastly, phone your mates, they'll be pleased to hear from you and overjoyed that you aren't asking for a lift home, or for bail.

Tip 98

Holding Your Baby

You may have worried the whole time during the pregnancy that you would be incapable of holding your baby without dropping her. It's simply not true. Take a seat, accept the little bundle of joy and within five minutes you'll think you've been doing it for years. So, I know you've been looking – whose ears has she got?

Tip 99

Wetting the Baby's Head

It may not be the wild stag night do that you had in mind, but try, try, try to arrange a night out with your friends while your partner is still in hospital. It really will be your last chance in ages; and although you'll be ecstatic, elated and exhausted all at the same time, raising a glass or two to your newborn child has got to be one of the most wonderful feelings in the world.

Tip 100

The New Family

Ensure that someone takes a photo of the three of you together, as soon as possible. It's so easy to take a hundred photos of a newborn, but how much more poignant to have you all together for the first time. And that means you too, you big hairy hunk.

Words of praise for
The Bloke's Guide to Pregnancy

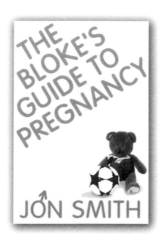

'Excellent advice and information on everything – from options on the type of birth and medical interventions, to being the partner's voice during the birth.' ***Relate Magazine***

'Jon Smith gives his lowdown on what men should expect over the happy but stressful nine-month countdown.' ***Daily Express***

'Right-on.' ***YOU* magazine, *Mail on Sunday***

Available from December 2006

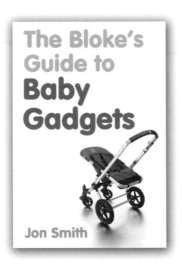

Any 'Dad-to-be' may not get excited about ante-natal classes or the intricacies of each trimester, but he definitely will care about the gear. Covering everything from buggies to wipe warmers, mobiles to wheelie bugs, The Bloke's Guide to Baby Gadgets reviews every contraption, gizmo, device and thingamajig in the market today.

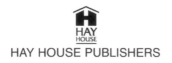

We hope you enjoyed this Hay House book.
If you would like to receive a free catalogue featuring additional
Hay House books and products, or if you would like information
about the Hay Foundation, please contact:

Hay House UK Ltd

292B Kensal Rd • London W10 5BE
Tel: (44) 20 8962 1230; Fax: (44) 20 8962 1239
www.hayhouse.co.uk

***

Published and distributed in the United States of America by:
Hay House, Inc. • PO Box 5100 • Carlsbad, CA 92018-5100
Tel: (1) 760 431 7695 or (800) 654 5126;
Fax: (1) 760 431 6948 or (800) 650 5115
www.hayhouse.com

Published and distributed in Australia by:
Hay House Australia Ltd • 18/36 Ralph St • Alexandria NSW 2015
Tel: (61) 2 9669 4299; Fax: (61) 2 9669 4144
www.hayhouse.com.au

Published and distributed in the Republic of South Africa by:
Hay House SA (Pty) Ltd • PO Box 990 • Witkoppen 2068
Tel/Fax: (27) 11 706 6612 • orders@psdprom.co.za

Distributed in Canada by:
Raincoast • 9050 Shaughnessy St • Vancouver, BC V6P 6E5
Tel: (1) 604 323 7100; Fax: (1) 604 323 2600

***

Sign up via the Hay House UK website to receive the Hay House
online newsletter and stay informed about what's going on with
your favourite authors. You'll receive bimonthly announcements
about discounts and offers, special events, product highlights,
free excerpts, giveaways, and more!
www.hayhouse.co.uk